About the NCCN Guidelines for Patients®

National Comprehensive Cancer Network®

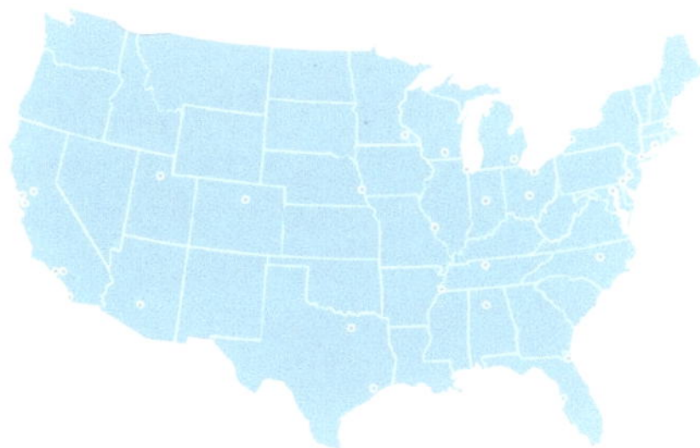

Did you know that top cancer centers across the United States work together to improve cancer care? This alliance of leading cancer centers is called the National Comprehensive Cancer Network® (NCCN®).

Cancer care is always changing. NCCN develops evidence-based cancer care recommendations used by health care providers worldwide. These frequently updated recommendations are the NCCN Clinical Practice Guidelines in Oncology (NCCN Guidelines®). The NCCN Guidelines for Patients plainly explain these expert recommendations for people with cancer and caregivers.

These NCCN Guidelines for Patients are based on the NCCN Clinical Practice Guidelines in Oncology (NCCN Guidelines®) for Soft Tissue Sarcoma, Version 1.2025 — May 2, 2025.

Learn how the NCCN Guidelines for Patients are developed
NCCN.org/patient-guidelines-process

View the NCCN Guidelines for Patients free online
NCCN.org/patientguidelines

Find an NCCN Cancer Center near you
NCCN.org/cancercenters

Connect with us YouTube

Supporters

NCCN Guidelines for Patients are supported by funding from the NCCN Foundation®

NCCN Foundation gratefully acknowledges the following corporate supporters for helping to make available these NCCN Guidelines for Patients:
Aadi Bioscience; and SpringWorks Therapeutics, Inc.

NCCN independently adapts, updates, and hosts the NCCN Guidelines for Patients. Our corporate supporters do not participate in the development of the NCCN Guidelines for Patients and are not responsible for the content and recommendations contained therein.

Additional support has been provided by

Dottie Shead, MS

Sarcoma Foundation of America (SFA) improves outcomes for people diagnosed with sarcoma by funding and advancing research, educating and providing resources for people diagnosed with sarcoma, advocating on behalf of the community, and growing awareness. As the largest private funder of research in the sarcoma community, SFA has provided over $26 million to support more than 230 grants at 127 institutions in 13 countries. SFA is also the most visible and comprehensive sarcoma patient advocacy organization representing all subtypes. For more information, visit curesarcoma.org.

To make a gift or learn more, visit online or email

NCCNFoundation.org/Donate

PatientGuidelines@NCCN.org

Contents

NCCN Foundation seeks to support the millions of patients and their families affected by a cancer diagnosis by funding and distributing NCCN Guidelines for Patients. NCCN Foundation is also committed to advancing cancer treatment by funding the nation's promising doctors at the center of innovation in cancer research. For more details and the full library of patient and caregiver resources, visit NCCN.org/patients.

National Comprehensive Cancer Network (NCCN) and NCCN Foundation
3025 Chemical Road, Suite 100, Plymouth Meeting, PA 19462 USA

1 About soft tissue sarcoma

You or someone you know has soft tissue sarcoma. This is a scary and stressful time in your life. What is soft tissue sarcoma? This chapter explains what it is and how it's treated.

What is soft tissue sarcoma?

Soft tissue sarcoma (pronounced saar·KOH·muh) is a disease where cells in the soft tissue multiply and grow out of control. Most sarcomas are a form of cancer, but there are certain types of benign tumors (not cancer) that can also be categorized as sarcoma.

Soft tissue is a general term that includes almost any tissue in the body that isn't bone. Skin, fat, muscle, tendons, ligaments, nerves, blood vessels, and lymph vessels are all soft tissues. Soft tissues connect with other tissues and support the organs in the body.

Soft tissue sarcoma

Soft tissue includes fat, muscles, nerves, tendons, blood and lymph vessels, and other supportive tissues of the body.

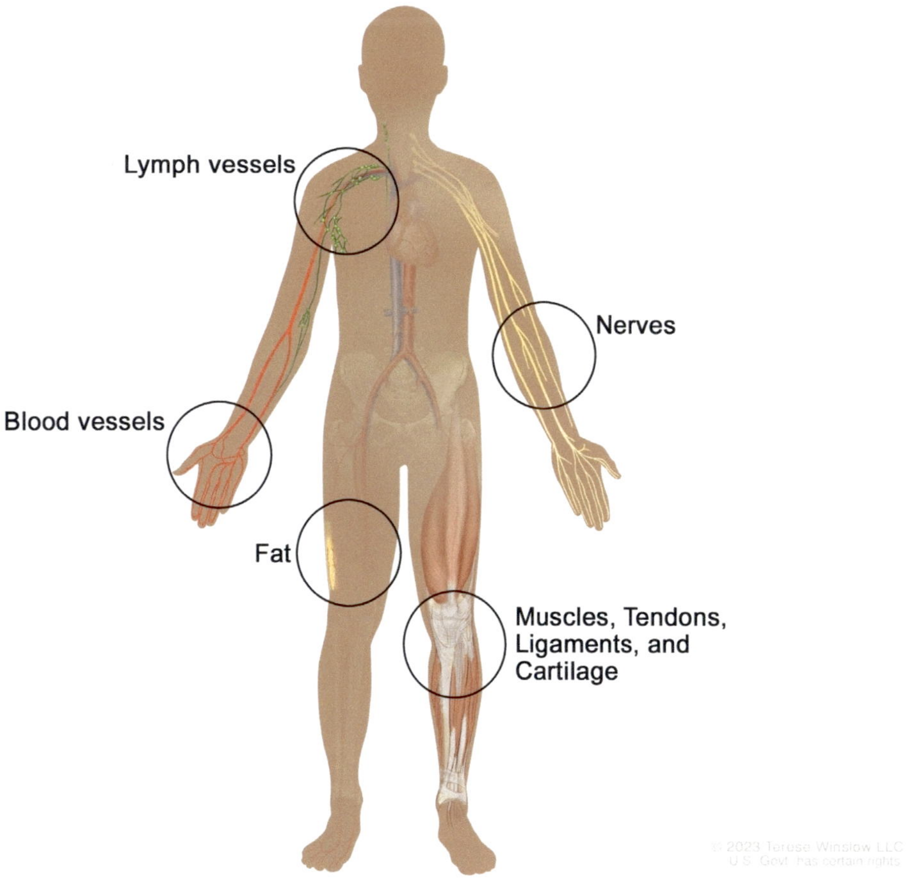

Soft tissue sarcoma is a cancer that develops in these tissues. Cancer occurs when something goes wrong with the natural cell process, causing some soft tissue cells to become cancer cells.

Cancer cells don't behave like normal cells. They develop genetic changes that allow them to multiply and make many more cancer cells. The cancer cells crowd out and overwhelm normal cells.

Cancer cells also survive much longer than normal cells do. They can replace many normal cells and cause organs to stop working properly. This can end up harming the body.

Cancer cells can also spread outside the affected soft tissues and form tumors in other areas of the body. This is called metastatic soft tissue sarcoma.

The other, less common types of sarcomas are bone or cartilage sarcoma, such as osteosarcoma or chondrosarcoma. More information about osteosarcoma and other bone sarcomas can be found in the *NCCN Guidelines for Patients: Bone Cancer*, available at NCCN.org/patientguidelines and on the NCCN Patient Guides for Cancer app.

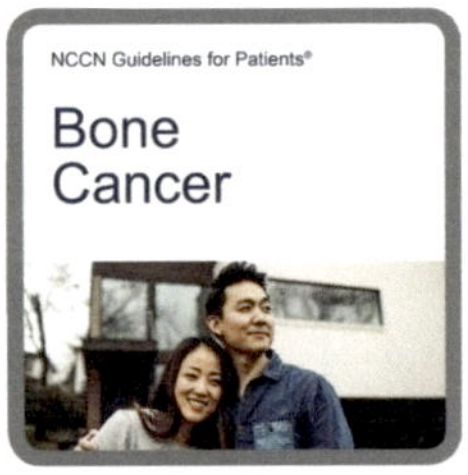

Why you should read this book

Making decisions about cancer care can be stressful. You may need to make tough decisions under pressure about complex choices.

The NCCN Guidelines for Patients are trusted by patients and providers. They clearly explain current care recommendations made by respected experts in the field. Recommendations are based on the latest research and practices at leading cancer centers.

Cancer care is not the same for everyone. By following expert recommendations for your situation, you are more likely to improve your care and have better outcomes as a result. Use this book as your guide to find the information you need to make important decisions.

What causes soft tissue sarcoma?

Cancer researchers don't know what causes soft tissue cells to grow out of control (become cancerous). But several factors are linked to a higher risk of soft tissue sarcoma. These are called risk factors. A risk factor is anything that increases your chance of getting cancer.

Risk factors don't necessarily cause soft tissue sarcoma. You can have cancer without those factors. These are the main risk factors for soft tissue sarcoma:

- Exposure to certain chemicals (pesticides and herbicides, for example)
- Previous radiation exposure from cancer treatment (this is called radiation-associated sarcoma)
- Hereditary or genetic syndromes (see more information in Chapter 2)

How are soft tissue sarcomas treated?

For soft tissue sarcomas that have not spread to other areas of the body, surgery is the main form of treatment. Sometimes radiation or chemotherapy is used. For soft tissue sarcoma that has spread, chemotherapy is used.

Soft tissue sarcomas are not common, and some are so rare that cancer care providers don't have set ways to treat them. Many cancer care providers don't have the background to diagnose or treat these tumors. Find out more about diagnosis in *Chapter 2: Testing for soft tissue sarcoma*.

Soft tissue sarcomas in this book are divided into:

- Sarcomas in the limbs, torso, head, or neck
- Sarcomas inside the abdomen
- Desmoid tumors
- Rhabdomyosarcoma (RMS)
- Atypical lipomatous tumor (ALT)/well-differentiated liposarcoma (WDLS)

Experts from NCCN have written treatment guidelines for soft tissue sarcomas, including those explained in this book. Looking at these treatments can help you understand how they work, especially if your doctor recommends one for you. Read more about treatment in *Chapter 3: Types of treatment*.

If your sarcoma is not mentioned in this book, try to find a treatment center or hospital with experts who have experience in your type of soft tissue sarcoma.

If you don't live close to a treatment center, experts can provide you with a treatment plan and coordinate with your local health care providers. This would allow you to receive the best care possible closer to home.

Certain types of treatments, such as clinical trials or special kinds of radiation therapy, may only be available at specialized treatment centers or hospitals.

What can you do to get the best care?

Advocate for yourself. You have an important role to play in your care. In fact, you're more likely to get the care you want by asking questions and making shared decisions with your care team.

The NCCN Guidelines for Patients will help you understand cancer care. With better understanding, you'll be more prepared to discuss your care with your team and share your concerns. Many people feel more satisfied when they play an active role in their care.

You may not know what to ask your care team. That's common. Each chapter in this book ends with an important section called *Questions to ask*. These suggested questions will help you get more information on all aspects of your care.

Take the next step and keep reading to learn what is the best care for you!

Adolescents and young adults (AYAs) with cancer have unique medical, mental, emotional, and social concerns.

The focus of this guide is treatment of soft tissue sarcoma in adults. AYAs with soft tissue sarcoma have age-specific problems and needs. See the *NCCN Guidelines for Patients: Adolescent and Young Adult Cancer*, available at NCCN.org/patientguidelines and on the NCCN Patient Guides for Cancer app.

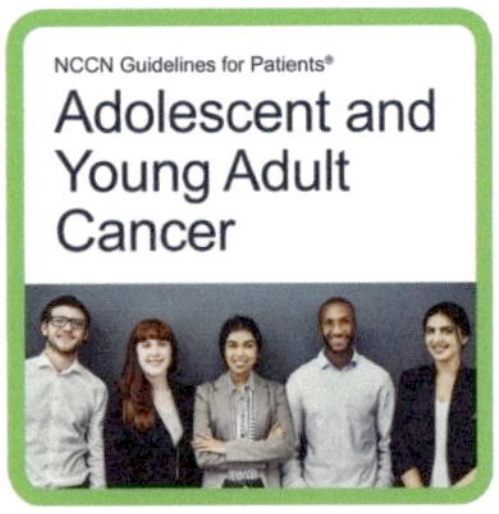

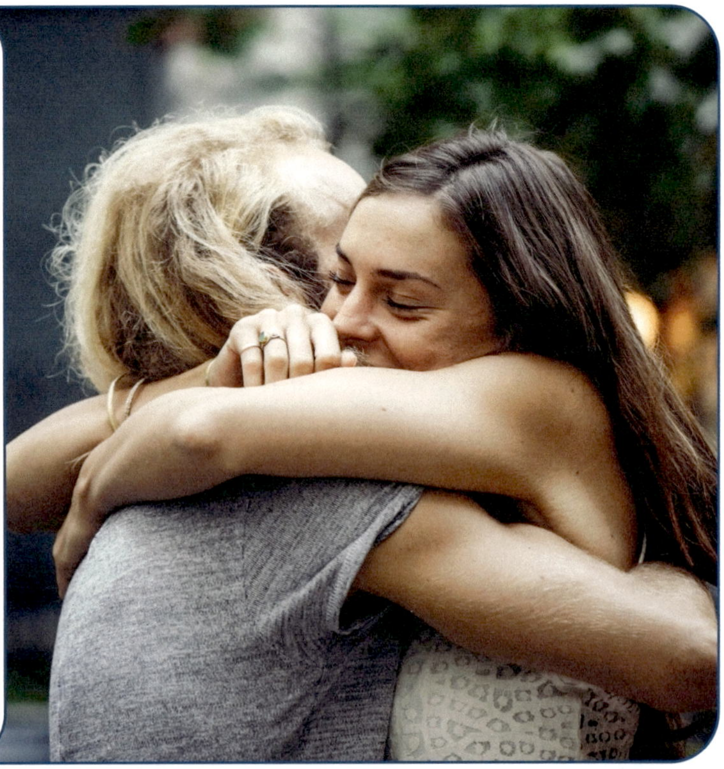

2

Testing for soft tissue sarcoma

Testing for suspected soft tissue sarcoma starts with imaging scans and a biopsy. Other testing is based on the location of the tumor and your health history.

Imaging

Imaging tests take pictures of areas inside the body. They can show the primary (first) tumor and other possible areas of cancer. The imaging tests used most often for soft tissue sarcoma are computed tomography (CT) and magnetic resonance imaging (MRI).

CT and MRI

CT, also called a CAT scan, takes many x-rays of the same body part from different angles. The images are combined using a computer to make a series of cross-sectional images of the inside of the body.

MRI uses radio waves and powerful magnets to take pictures of areas inside the body. Unlike CT, it does not use radiation. If you have any metal in your body, tell your radiation tech before having an MRI, as MRIs may not be safe for you.

The choice of CT versus MRI depends on the type and location of the tumor. For example, MRI is preferred for tumors in the brain, spine, liver, and extremities. Both CT and MRI can provide details about the size of the tumor and how close it is to nearby organs, nerves, and blood vessels.

A radiologist is an expert at interpreting medical scans. They will review the images

CT scan

A CT scan is a more detailed type of x-ray. It is painless and noninvasive. CT takes many images from different angles. A computer combines the images to make 3D pictures.

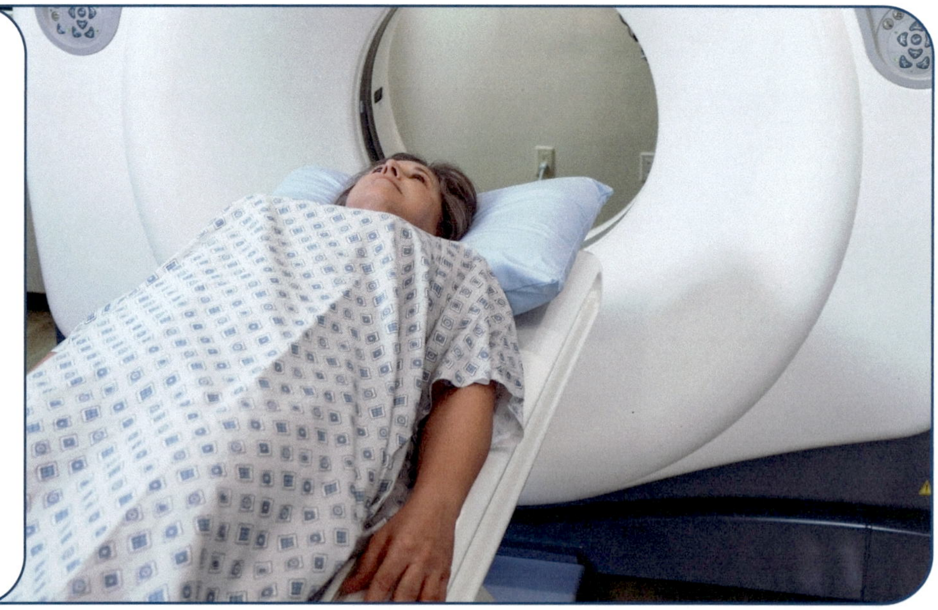

and write a report. The radiologist will send this report to your health care provider, who will discuss the results with you. Depending on what they see, the radiologist may suggest that you have another or a different type of imaging scan.

Contrast

Before or during a CT or MRI, you might be given a contrast agent. Contrast is a substance that changes how tissues look in pictures.

Tell your care team if you've had a reaction to contrast in the past. Contrast might not be used if you have a serious allergy or if your kidneys don't work well.

PET

Positron emission tomography (PET) scans use a radioactive substance called a tracer or isotope. This substance accumulates in places that use a lot of energy in your body.

Most cancer cells, including sarcoma cells, use much more energy than normal cells and show up as bright spots on PET scans. However, not all bright spots are cancer. Not all cancers appear on PET scans.

PET is usually combined with CT scans to provide additional helpful information.

Team approach to care

Treating soft tissue sarcoma takes a team approach. Treatment planning should involve a team of doctors from different fields of medicine who have experience in soft tissue sarcoma. Some members of your care team will be with you throughout treatment, while others will only be there for parts of it. Get to know your care team and help them get to know you.

- **A pathologist** diagnoses cancer by studying cells and tissues under a microscope.
- **A diagnostic radiologist** reads the results of x-rays and other imaging tests such as an MRI or CT scan.
- **An orthopedic surgical oncologist** performs operations to remove soft tissue and bone sarcomas that involve the pelvis, spine, and extremities. They perform limb salvage surgery and reconstruct bones after a bone tumor is removed.
- **A surgical oncologist** performs operations to remove cancer from the torso, abdomen, and sometimes the extremities.
- **A medical oncologist** treats cancer in adults using systemic drug therapy, which goes through the body. This person often leads the overall treatment team.
- **A radiation oncologist** prescribes and plans radiation therapy to treat cancer.

Biopsy

After imaging tests, your health care provider will usually order or perform a biopsy. This involves removing a sample of the tumor and testing it for cancer.

The preferred type of biopsy for soft tissue sarcoma is a core needle biopsy. It removes tissue with a wide, hollow needle.

Another type, called an incisional biopsy or open biopsy, removes a small amount of tissue through a cut in the skin or body. Sometimes, health care providers may perform a biopsy using a thinner needle, called fine-needle aspiration.

Most soft tissue sarcomas are deep within the body. For these tumors, biopsies are guided using imaging, such as an ultrasound or CT. Image-guided needle biopsies are usually needed for tumors in the chest, abdomen, pelvis, and abdominal organs.

If your health care provider believes that your tumor is close to the skin, they may perform a biopsy without imaging guidance.

Testing the tumor sample

A pathologist is an expert in examining tissues and cells to diagnose disease. After examining the tissues and cells with a microscope, the pathologist writes a summary of the results. This is called a pathology report.

Pathologists often perform other tests to see if the tumor cells have specific genes or proteins. This is often necessary to diagnose the tumor type. This may also help refine which treatment is better for your tumor type.

Because not all pathologists are familiar with every type of soft tissue sarcoma, you should ensure that your tests are reviewed at an experienced center. Ask questions about your biopsy results and what they mean for your treatment. You can also ask for your tissue samples to be analyzed at a different medical center for a second opinion.

Genetic tests and genetic syndromes

Certain genetic syndromes increase the risk of developing soft tissue sarcoma. Changes in different genes (called mutations) cause each of these genetic syndromes.

You inherit your genes from your parents. In hereditary or genetic syndromes, your siblings, your parents' siblings, and your grandparents often have the same mutation.

Testing for gene mutations that cause these syndromes may help treat soft tissue sarcoma and monitor you or your family members for cancers.

Share what you know about your personal health and family history with your care team. If your health care provider thinks you may have a genetic syndrome that is causing your cancer, you may benefit from genetic testing.

Testing should be carried out by a pathologist who's experienced in genetic testing techniques. A genetic counselor may speak with you about the results. A genetic counselor is an expert who has special training in genetic diseases.

The following syndromes are genetic and can be risk factors for soft tissue sarcoma:

Carney-Stratakis syndrome

This rare inherited disorder causes gastrointestinal stromal tumors (GIST) and paragangliomas. Paragangliomas are tumors that form in embryonic (embryo) nervous tissues in the head, neck, and torso. They are usually benign (not cancer).

FAP

People with familial adenomatous polyposis (FAP) have a gene mutation in a tumor suppressor gene called adenomatous polyposis coli. This syndrome causes many polyps to form in the colon and rectum. These polyps start as noncancerous growths, but over time they can turn into cancer.

Gardner syndrome

FAP has a related syndrome, called Gardner syndrome. In addition to bowel polyps, those with Gardner syndrome have abnormal bony growths, skin tumors, and soft tissue tumors.

Your care team will gather information to determine if you're likely to have Gardner syndrome or FAP. Both are associated with desmoid tumors, which aren't cancerous (they don't spread to other parts of the body) but grow aggressively. If you're diagnosed with a desmoid tumor, your family history should be looked at closely.

Hereditary retinoblastoma

Retinoblastoma is cancer in the retina (the light-sensitive nerve tissue at the back of the eye). It's most common in children under the age of 5.

Retinoblastoma may be hereditary or nonhereditary. The hereditary form increases the risk of leiomyosarcoma and bone sarcoma.

Li-Fraumeni syndrome

Families with Li-Fraumeni syndrome have a mutation in the *TP53* gene. This gene helps control the repair or survival of damaged cells.

Families with Li-Fraumeni syndrome have a history of sarcoma, breast cancer, tumors in the adrenal glands (where adrenaline is made), and some brain tumors. People with a personal and/or family history that suggests Li-Fraumeni syndrome should be considered for further genetic testing.

Lynch syndrome

Lynch syndrome is also called hereditary non-polyposis colorectal cancer, or HNPCC for short. Those born with Lynch syndrome are at high risk of developing colorectal cancer and some other cancers, particularly endometrial and ovarian cancer.

While not common (less than 1 percent of people have Lynch syndrome), it can also increase the risk of soft tissue sarcoma.

Neurofibromatosis

This rare genetic condition causes tumors to grow on nerves. These tumors are usually malignant peripheral nerve sheath tumors, also known as MPNSTs. About 5 out of 100 people (5 percent) with neurofibromatosis will also develop soft tissue sarcoma.

What's next?

After the type of soft tissue sarcoma has been identified, you'll undergo treatment. The next few chapters focus on the types of treatments available and which ones apply to which body areas.

Key points

- Testing for suspected soft tissue sarcoma starts with imaging and a biopsy.
- A core needle biopsy is generally preferred for diagnosing soft tissue sarcoma.
- MRI and CT scans provide details about the size and location of the tumor. Imaging is usually done before biopsy.
- Other testing is based on the location of the tumor and your health history.
- Your health care provider might refer you for genetic testing to learn more about your cancer.

Questions to ask

- Will my insurance pay for all of the tests you're recommending?
- Do I need to do anything to prepare for testing?
- Should I bring someone with me to the appointments?
- Where do I go for testing, and how long will it take?
- Is this treatment option a standard of care or a clinical trial?

3
Types of treatment

Your treatment options will depend on the location and type of soft tissue sarcoma. This chapter describes surgery, radiation therapy, and other commonly used treatments.

Treatment can be local, can work throughout the body ("systemic"), or can be a combination of both. Local therapy treats the tumor directly. Surgery and radiation therapy are local therapies. Chemotherapy, targeted therapy, and immunotherapy are systemic drug therapies.

Goals of care

Before deciding on treatment, you and your providers need to establish the goals of care.

For many people, the chance to not have the tumor return is often the priority. But there are other goals of care to consider, such as maintaining quality of life or living without side effects of treatment.

Surgery

Surgery is the main treatment for sarcoma that has not spread. The method and extent of surgery for sarcoma depend on the tumor's location and size, and whether it involves nearby body parts.

Imaging tests are used to determine if your cancer can be removed with surgery or can't be safely removed with surgery. Unremovable tumors often involve other critical body structures. In some cases, the tumor is so extensive that surgery can't remove the whole tumor.

Your surgeon will use the pre-surgery imaging studies to plan the operation and will explain what to expect for recovery afterward.
The surgeon will attempt to remove all the sarcoma, but sometimes tumor cells that could not be seen during the operation are left behind.

The goal of surgery is to remove all the cancer. To do so, the tumor is removed along with a rim of normal-looking tissue around its edge. This rim of normal-looking tissue is called the surgical margin.

A clear or negative margin is the best result. It means that there was a layer of normal tissue surrounding the entire tumor that was removed. It also means there is a decreased chance that any cancer cells were left behind.

If all the visible tumor is removed, but the pathologist finds cancer cells at the margin, it's called a microscopically positive margin.

Sometimes, however, it's not possible to safely remove the sarcoma with a cancer-free margin.

You also might have more than one surgery. You might also have a temporary wound drain to prevent fluid from collecting in the body after surgery. A wound drain is a tube connected to a surgical wound that allows fluid to drain out into a reservoir outside of the body.

Limb-sparing surgery

When surgery involves a limb (an arm or a leg), the goal is to have a functional or working limb after the tumor is removed. This is called limb-sparing surgery. Most surgeries to remove sarcomas in a limb use limb-sparing surgery.

Rehabilitation before or after surgery will likely be part of a limb-sparing treatment plan. Occupational therapy helps with daily life skills. Physical therapy helps your body move and function.

After surgery to remove a sarcoma, some people may suffer from lymphedema, or swelling in the limb. This can worsen if radiation is also a part of the treatment. Lymphedema therapists can provide techniques and compression garments that can help reduce this swelling.

Amputation

Amputation is the removal of a limb or other body part. A surgeon who is an expert in soft tissue sarcoma should be consulted to determine if amputation is necessary or if the limb can remain, if possible.

Rehabilitation, such as physical and occupational therapy, will be part of this treatment. Seek a peer support group to connect with others who have experienced the loss of a limb. This will aid in your recovery and help you to maintain an active lifestyle.

Surgical margin

The tumor will be removed, along with some normal-looking tissue around its rim. The normal-looking tissue is called the surgical margin. The surgical margin will be tested for cancer. Postoperative therapy is based on if there is cancer in the margins.

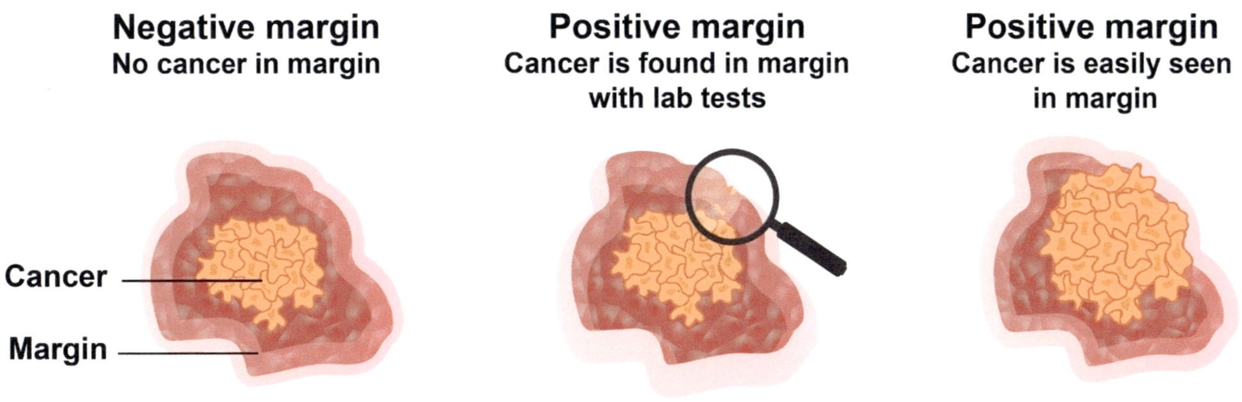

Metastasectomy

A metastasectomy is surgery to remove one or more distant tumors (a metastasis or metastases) that have spread from the original tumor. This is not the same surgery as a mastectomy, which is the removal of a breast. A common organ for metastasectomy in soft tissue sarcoma is the lung.

Whether you can have a metastasectomy depends on the tumor's location, the amount of tissue that needs to be removed, and your overall health. Metastasectomy is more likely to be an option when the primary tumor can be completely removed and there are only a few small distant tumors that can be safely removed by surgery.

A metastasectomy may be done at the same time as surgery to remove the primary tumor. Or it may be done during a separate operation. The amount of time needed for the surgery and recovery depends on many factors. Some factors include the size, location of the metastases, and the type of surgery needed.

Palliative surgery

Surgery may also be used to relieve symptoms caused by cancer or to extend life. This is called palliative surgery.

For example, you could receive a metastasectomy to relieve pain caused by a tumor pressing on a nerve.

Debulking surgery (removing part, but not all of the tumor) is sometimes done as palliative surgery.

Radiation therapy

Radiation therapy uses high-energy x-rays, gamma rays, protons, or other sources to kill cancer cells. It's given alone or with chemotherapy over a fixed period of time.

Radiation may be used to sterilize the tumor before surgery. This can make it harder to remove the tumor, but lowers the chances of the tumor coming back. Radiation may also interfere with healing after surgery.

Radiation is sometimes given to kill leftover cancer cells after surgery. This may be recommended if not all the cancer was removed during surgery, or if there is a high risk of it growing back.

When given after surgery, radiation may lead to increased scarring or stiffness, called fibrosis. Fibrosis can reduce movement in the affected limb.

Radiation can also be used during surgery, called intraoperative radiation therapy. Or it can be used to ease pain or discomfort caused by the tumor. This is called palliative radiation therapy.

The 2 main types of radiation treatment are explained next. The method used depends on the size and type of sarcoma and the goal of treatment.

External radiation therapy

External beam radiation therapy (EBRT) uses a machine outside the body to aim radiation precisely at the tumor inside the body. Types of EBRT used to treat soft tissue sarcoma include:

- **Intensity-modulated radiation therapy** is an advanced radiation technique that uses many small beams of different strengths.
- **Image-guided radiation therapy** helps guide the radiation beam during treatment. Tumors can shift slightly within the body and can change shape and size between and during treatment visits. This technique can improve how well intensity-modulated radiation therapy targets the tumor.
- **Stereotactic body radiation therapy** uses high-energy radiation beams to treat metastatic tumors in five or fewer sessions.
- **Proton radiation therapy** uses streams of particles called protons to kill tumor cells and may reduce the amount of radiation damage to nearby healthy tissue.
- **Intraoperative radiation therapy** uses radiation treatment aimed directly at the tumor during surgery.

Internal radiation therapy

In internal radiation therapy, a radiation source is placed inside or next to the tumor. This is also called brachytherapy. Internal radiation therapy may be used alone or with EBRT. When used with EBRT, it's called a brachytherapy boost.

Radiation therapy

Radiation therapy uses high-energy radiation from x-rays, gamma rays, protons, and other sources to kill cancer cells and shrink tumors. It is also used to treat pain.

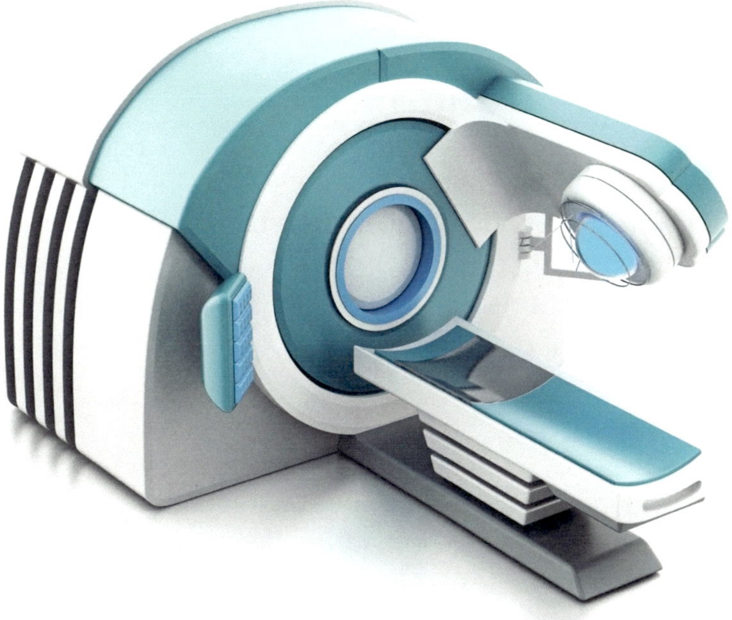

Low-dose-rate internal radiation therapy
Low-dose-rate internal radiation therapy uses thin, hollow needles to place radioactive "seeds" into the tumor. The seeds are about the size of a grain of rice. They are guided into the tumor with imaging.

The seeds stay in the tumor and give a low dose of radiation for a few months. The radiation travels a very short distance. This allows for a large amount of radiation within a small area (the tumor), while sparing nearby healthy tissue.

Over time, the seeds stop radiating but will stay in your body permanently.

High-dose-rate internal radiation therapy
High-dose-rate internal radiation therapy involves thin needles inserted into the tumor. These needles are then attached to tubes called catheters. Radiation is delivered through these catheters.

After treatment, the needles and catheters are removed.

Other local treatments

Some of the following therapies are used together with surgery or radiation therapy. Ablation can be performed during surgery, for example. This ensures that more of the tumor can be removed, if possible.

Isolated limb infusion

Isolated limb infusion is used to treat sarcoma of the limb. It involves delivering anti-cancer drugs directly into an arm or leg.

During surgery, the flow of blood is stopped for a short time while the drugs are injected into the blood of the limb. This limits the effect of chemotherapy on the rest of the body.

This option should only be done at centers or hospitals with experience in regional limb therapy.

Thermal ablation

Thermal ablation uses extreme cold or extreme heat to destroy cancer cells. It can destroy small tumors with little harm to nearby tissue.

A similar procedure you may have already had is freezing off a mole or wart, done by your dermatologist or at home with an over-the-counter freezing solution. The principle is the same.

There are 2 types of thermal ablation used to destroy cancer cells:

- Cryotherapy kills cancer cells by freezing them with a very cold substance.
- Radiofrequency ablation kills cancer cells by heating them with high-energy radio waves.

Both types use a special needle, called a probe, which is inserted into the tumor. With cryotherapy, a gas is passed through the probe to freeze the tumor and destroy it. With radiofrequency ablation, the probe emits radio waves to heat the tumor and destroy it.

The probe can be guided into place with a CT scan, ultrasound, or other imaging tests. The probe is removed when treatment is done.

Embolization

All solid tumors need blood to live and grow. Embolization treats tumors by cutting off their blood supply. It can be used before surgery to remove a tumor.

A catheter is inserted into an artery and guided to the tumor. Once in place, beads are inserted to block the blood flow. In chemoembolization, the beads are coated with chemotherapy. In radioembolization, the beads are radioactive.

Systemic drug therapy

Cancer treatment that affects the whole body is called systemic therapy. Chemotherapy and chemoradiation, targeted therapy, and immunotherapy are types of systemic drug therapy.

Many systemic therapies are drugs that are injected into a vein or under the skin with a needle. Others are taken by mouth as a pill.

Chemotherapy

Chemotherapy kills fast-growing cells throughout the body, including cancer cells and normal cells. Many chemotherapy drugs are available to treat soft tissue sarcoma. More than one drug may be used.

Most chemotherapy is given in cycles. One cycle usually includes several treatment days followed by days or weeks of rest. This allows the body to recover between treatments. Cycles vary in length depending on which drugs are used. The number of treatment days per cycle and the total number of cycles given also vary.

Chemoradiation

Treatment that combines chemotherapy with radiation therapy is called chemoradiation. Chemotherapy may improve how well radiation works, and that's why they are sometimes used together. It's a combination of systemic and local therapies.

Targeted therapy

Targeted therapy is drug therapy that focuses on specific or unique features of cancer cells. For example, if your genetic test says that your tumor has an *NTRK* gene fusion, you might be treated with entrectinib (Rozlytrek).

Targeted therapy isn't used for every sarcoma. It might be used alone or with chemotherapy.

Immunotherapy

The immune system is the body's natural defense against infection and disease. It's a complex network of cells, tissues, and organs. Immunotherapy increases the activity of your immune system. By doing so, it improves your body's ability to find and destroy cancer cells.

Pembrolizumab (Keytruda), ipilimumab (Yervoy), and nivolumab (Opdivo) are types of immunotherapy.

Clinical trials

You may also be able to obtain treatment through a clinical trial.

A clinical trial is a type of medical research study. After being developed and tested in a lab, potential new ways of fighting cancer need to be studied in people.

If found to be safe and effective in a clinical trial, a drug, device, or treatment approach may be approved by the U.S. Food and Drug Administration (FDA).

Everyone with cancer should carefully consider all of the treatment options available for their cancer type, including standard treatments and clinical trials. Talk to your health care provider about whether a clinical trial may make sense for you.

Phases

Most cancer clinical trials focus on treatment and are done in phases.

- **Phase 1** trials study the safety and side effects of an investigational drug or treatment approach.
- **Phase 2** trials study how well the drug or approach works against a specific type of cancer.
- **Phase 3** trials test the drug or approach against a standard treatment. If the results are good, it may be approved by the FDA.
- **Phase 4** trials study the safety and benefit of an FDA-approved treatment.

Finding a clinical trial

In the United States

NCCN Cancer Centers
NCCN.org/cancercenters

The National Cancer Institute (NCI)
cancer.gov/about-cancer/treatment/clinical-trials/search

Worldwide

The U.S. National Library of Medicine (NLM)
clinicaltrials.gov

Need help finding a clinical trial?

NCI's Cancer Information Service (CIS)
1.800.4.CANCER (1.800.422.6237)
cancer.gov/contact

Who can enroll?

It depends on the clinical trial's rules, called eligibility criteria. The rules may be about age, cancer type and stage, treatment history, or general health. They ensure that participants are alike in specific ways and that the trial is as safe as possible for the participants.

Informed consent

Clinical trials are managed by a research team. This group of experts will review the study with you in detail, including its purpose and the risks and benefits of joining. All of this information is also provided in an informed consent form. Read the form carefully and ask questions before signing it. Take time to discuss it with people you trust. Keep in mind that you can leave and seek treatment outside of the clinical trial at any time.

Will I get a placebo?

Placebos (inactive versions of real medicines) are almost never used alone in cancer clinical trials. It's common to receive either a placebo with a standard treatment or a new drug with a standard treatment. You'll be informed, verbally and in writing, if a placebo is part of a clinical trial before you enroll.

Are clinical trials free?

There is no fee to enroll in a clinical trial. The study sponsor pays for research-related costs, including the study drug. But you may need to pay for other services, like transportation or childcare, due to extra appointments. During the trial, you'll continue to receive standard cancer care. This care is often covered by insurance.

What's next?

The next few chapters discuss specific sarcoma treatments by body location or tumor type. Read on to learn more about what treatments are right for you.

Key points

- When possible, surgery is often the preferred treatment for soft tissue sarcoma if it has not spread.
- In the best cases, surgery removes the tumor along with some normal-looking tissue around it (the surgical margin).
- Radiation therapy is a local treatment that is often used before or after surgery to lower the risk of the tumor growing back after surgery.
- Radiation therapy can also be used alone as a main (primary) treatment, or to relieve pain and discomfort caused by the tumor(s).
- Other local treatments include isolated limb infusion, thermal ablation, and embolization.
- Chemotherapy, targeted therapy, and immunotherapy are types of systemic drug therapy.
- A clinical trial studies an investigative treatment to see how safe it is and how well it works.

Questions to ask

- Is a clinical trial an option for me?
- What will happen if I do nothing?
- Are you suggesting options other than what NCCN recommends? If yes, why?
- How do my age, sex, overall health, and other factors affect my options?
- What if I am pregnant or planning to become pregnant?

4

Sarcomas in the limbs, outer torso, head, or neck

This chapter describes treatment for soft tissue sarcomas in the arms, legs, outer torso, head, and neck. Treatment is based on the type and location of the tumor, as well as the cancer stage.

Many types of soft tissue sarcoma can form in the head, neck, limbs, or outer torso. The limbs include arms and legs. The outer torso includes the chest, back, buttocks, and abdomen.

Areas of the head and neck that could be affected include:

- Neck and throat
- Face and scalp
- Sinuses and nose
- Mouth and lips

Head and neck soft tissue sarcomas can be hard to deal with because of their location. The tumor is more likely to be close to bones, muscles, and nerves, making treatment difficult.

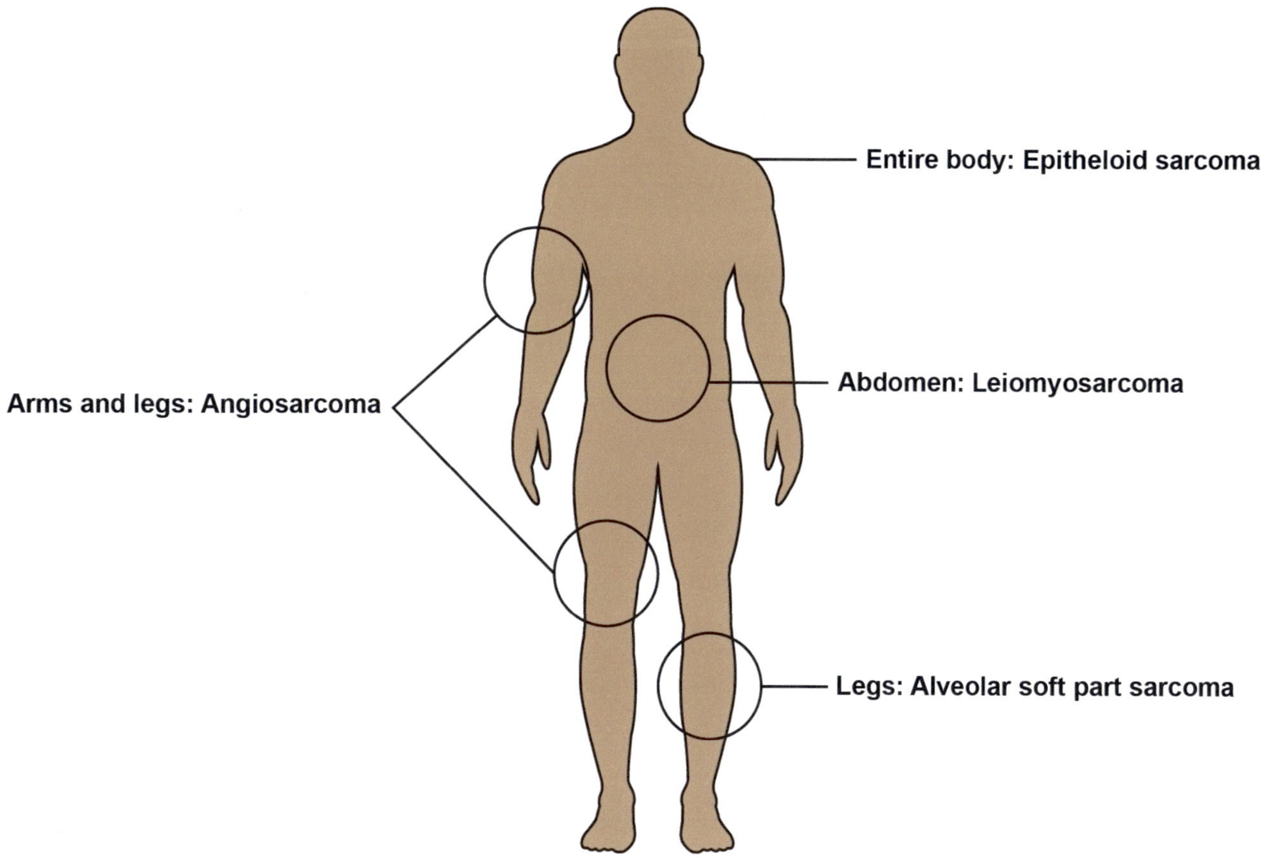

Some types of soft tissue sarcoma found in the limbs, outer torso, or head and neck (listed alphabetically) include:

- **Alveolar soft part sarcoma** begins in the soft tissue that surrounds organs and other tissues. It commonly occurs in the leg but can be found in the arms or torso.
- **Angiosarcoma** begins in the cells that line blood vessels or lymph vessels. These often occur in the limbs but can occur anywhere.
- **Atypical lipomatous tumors (ALT)/ well-differentiated liposarcoma (WDLS)** have cells that look like fat cells under a microscope. They tend to grow more slowly than poorly differentiated or undifferentiated cancer cells. When these grow in the extremities, they are not considered cancerous.
- **Dermatofibrosarcoma protuberans** occurs in the layer of tissue right under the skin. It starts as a nodule or thickening that grows slowly.
- **Epithelioid sarcoma** begins as a slow-growing, firm lump in the deep soft tissue or skin of the arms, hands, or fingers. It may also occur in the legs, torso, or head and neck. It's usually painless but tends to spread and return after treatment.
- **Leiomyosarcoma** is a cancer of smooth muscle cells that can arise almost anywhere in the body, most frequently in the abdomen.
- **Myxoid/round cell liposarcoma** begins in fat cells. It usually occurs in the thigh, but can be found in the outer torso and buttocks.

Staging soft tissue sarcoma

Your cancer care team will assign a stage to the cancer, usually with a number between 1 to 4. This helps your care team have a starting point for your treatment. It can also help you or your loved one, as the patient, understand the severity of the cancer diagnosis.

Stage 1A/1B sarcoma

In stage 1 sarcoma in the outer torso or limbs, the cancer has not spread to nearby lymph nodes or distant sites.

Stage 1 is further divided into stages 1A and 1B. These stages are both low-grade. This means the tumor isn't expected to grow quickly. The difference between the two is that stage 1A tumors can be monitored for some time before any treatment decision is made.

Surgery is the recommended treatment for stage 1A/1B sarcomas in these areas. If surgery is likely to leave tumor cells behind, treating the tumor with radiation therapy might be recommended before surgery.

The goal of surgery is to remove the sarcoma with no cancer in the surgical margin. However, to avoid cutting nerves and blood vessels, your surgeon may not be able to remove a large enough area. In this case, there is a higher chance that cancer cells will be left behind.

After the surgery, a pathologist will examine the surgical margin for cancer cells. If the sarcoma was completely removed (referred to as a "negative margin"), you can start follow-up care.

If not enough tissue around the sarcoma was removed (referred to as a "positive margin"), you may have a second surgery or radiation therapy.

Follow-up care

A physical exam is recommended every 3 to 6 months for the first 3 years after treatment. After that, visits are once per year.

Your health care provider will consider an imaging study after treatment to serve as your starting point. You may have periodic imaging of the surgery site. This is based on the risk of recurrence. If the tumor is in an area that's easy to access and examine (like the skin), imaging may not be needed.

If cancer is likely to spread to your lungs, your chest may be scanned periodically.

There is a risk of some physical disability with surgery to remove a soft tissue sarcoma. You should be evaluated for rehabilitation services. Such services include occupational and physical therapy.

Occupational therapy can help with daily life skills. Physical therapy helps your body move and function.

Stage 2, stage 3, and some stage 4 sarcomas

The following information applies to stage 2 and stage 3 sarcomas in the limbs or outer torso. It also applies to stage 4 sarcomas that have spread to nearby lymph nodes but not to other organs or tissues.

Treatment for these stages is based on whether surgery can be done. If the tumor can be safely removed and you'll have good use of the limb or area, it's called resectable or removable.

However, surgery might not be the first treatment. The tumor may be too large or removing it may limit the use of a limb or other body parts. Surgery may also cause health-related problems.

Other treatment is often given before or after surgery. Treatment before surgery may include chemoradiation, radiation therapy, or systemic drug therapy. The goal is to shrink the tumor beforehand so it's easier to remove during surgery.

Treatment after surgery is to "clean up" any remaining tumor cells that are left behind after surgery. The goal is to destroy any remaining tumor cells to reduce the chances of it returning.

Treatment is grouped into:

- Removable with good function
- Removable with poor function
- Unremovable

All "removable" options include surgery to remove the tumor.

Removable with good function

Stage 2 sarcoma
Surgery is the main treatment for removable stage 2 sarcomas. Radiation therapy may be given before or after surgery.

When given first, radiation can sterilize the surface of the tumor and improve the outcome of surgery. When given after surgery, radiation can eliminate any residual tumor cells left behind after surgery. Either form of radiation, given before or after surgery, can lower the risk of the cancer returning.

One downside is that when radiation therapy is done before surgery or before you've fully healed, it'll likely slow the healing process.

Stage 3 and some stage 4 sarcomas
If systemic drug therapy is planned, the choice of drug(s) will depend on the tumor type. Preferred systemic therapies for general soft tissue sarcoma are listed in **Guide 1**.

Preferred systemic drug therapies for specific tumor types are listed in **Guide 2**.

Possible treatment pathways for stage 3 and non-metastatic stage 4 sarcomas

Surgery	→	Radiation therapy or chemoradiation		
Radiation therapy	→	Surgery	→	Possible systemic drug therapy
Chemoradiation	→	Surgery	→	Possible systemic drug therapy
Systemic drug therapy	→	Surgery	→	Radiation therapy or chemoradiation

Guide 1
Preferred systemic drug therapies for general soft tissue sarcoma

Before or after surgery	• Doxorubicin, ifosfamide, mesna • Ifosfamide, epirubicin, mesna
First-line systemic drug therapy for advanced or metastatic disease	• Doxorubicin, dacarbazine • Doxorubicin, ifosfamide, mesna **Anthracycline-based regimens:** • Doxorubicin • Epirubicin • Ifosfamide, epirubicin, mesna • Liposomal doxorubicin **For *NTRK* gene fusion-positive sarcomas only:** • Larotrectinib • Entrectinib • Repotrectinib
Next-in-line therapy for advanced or metastatic disease	Anthracycline-based regimens, as listed above for first-line therapy, may be considered Eribulin (especially for liposarcoma) Gemcitabine and docetaxel Pazopanib Trabectedin (especially for liposarcoma and leiomyosarcoma) For *NTRK* gene fusion-positive sarcomas only: Repotrectinib

The systemic drug therapies listed in this guide are preferred for general soft tissue sarcoma. Other recommended drug therapies may be a better fit for you. Talk to your care team about your options.

Guide 2
Preferred systemic drug therapies for specific types of soft tissue sarcoma

Alveolar soft part sarcoma (ASPS)	Atezolizumab Pazopanib Pembrolizumab, with or without axitinib Sunitinib
Angiosarcoma	Anthracycline- or gemcitabine-based treatments recommended for general soft tissue sarcoma types Paclitaxel
DFSP with fibrosarcomatous transformation	Imatinib
Extraskeletal osteosarcoma	Usually treated with ifosfamide or platinum-based therapy (cisplatin/doxorubicin)
Dedifferentiated chordoma	Anthracycline- or gemcitabine-based treatments recommended for general soft tissue sarcoma types
Inflammatory myofibroblastic tumor (IMT) with *ALK* translocation	Alectinib Brigatinib Ceritinib Crizotinib Lorlatinib
Malignant PEComa	Albumin-bound sirolimus
Solitary fibrous tumor	Bevacizumab and temozolomide Pazopanib Sorafenib Sunitinib
Tenosynovial giant cell tumor/ pigmented villonodular synovitis	Pexidartinib
Recurrent angiomyolipoma, lymphangioleiomyomatosis	Sirolimus Temsirolimus Vimseltinib

The systemic drug therapies listed in this guide are preferred for specific types of soft tissue sarcoma. Other recommended options may be a better fit for you. Talk to your care team about them.

Unremovable or removable with poor function

Surgery may not be a first treatment option for stage 2, stage 3, or non-metastatic stage 4 sarcomas. This is often due to the tumor location and/or size. One of the following treatments is usually used first to shrink the tumor. If it works well, surgery may be possible.

- Radiation therapy
- Chemoradiation
- Systemic drug therapy
- Isolated limb infusion

After treatment, your health care providers will assess whether you're able to have surgery with good results.

Good results can include a surgical margin larger than 1 cm (the size of a pea or larger), cancer-free margins, and good use of your limb or other body part. This would mean that a tumor that was unremovable is now removable.

If the cancer becomes removable, see treatment information under *Removable with good function* on page 28.

If the cancer becomes removable but surgery would cause a loss of function, either radiation therapy or radical surgery (such as amputation) may be recommended.

If the cancer **remains unremovable** after treatment, options include:

- Radiation therapy (if the area was not already treated)
- Systemic drug therapy
- Observation (if you have no symptoms)
- Supportive care

If the cancer is causing symptoms such as making it difficult to use your arms or legs, palliative surgery or other supportive care may be recommended for relief.

Follow-up care

Your health care provider will order imaging when treatment ends. These scans will serve as a starting point to compare against future imaging results. You'll continue to get scans of the site where the primary tumor was. How often depends on how likely the cancer is to return.

Imaging of the chest is also recommended to look for cancer spread into the lungs.

A physical exam is recommended every 3 to 6 months for the first 3 years after treatment. For the following 2 years, visits are recommended every 6 months. After that, visits are once per year.

After 10 years, the risk of recurrence is very low. Talk to your treatment team about how long you should have follow-up care.

After surgery, you should also be evaluated for rehabilitation services. Such services include occupational and physical therapy. Occupational therapy can help with daily life skills. Physical therapy helps your body move and function.

Metastatic stage 4 sarcoma

Stage 4 soft tissue sarcoma of the limbs or outer torso has spread to distant areas or lymph nodes, or both. However, sarcomas are much less likely to spread to lymph nodes.

The following information applies to sarcomas found in distant areas when first diagnosed. Treatment depends on the extent of the cancer.

If there are only a few small metastatic tumors that can be treated with local therapies, treatment according to *Removable with good function* on page 28 is recommended. Your treatment team will consider the following options for treating metastatic tumors:

- Systemic drug therapy (see **Guides 1** and **2**)
- Surgery, with or without radiation therapy
- Stereotactic body radiation therapy
- Ablation methods
- Embolization (for tumors not in the lungs)
- Observation

Follow-up care

A physical exam is recommended every 2 to 6 months for the first 2 to 3 years after treatment. For the following 2 to 3 years, physicals are recommended every 6 months. After that, visits are once per year.

After 10 years, the risk of recurrence is very low. Talk to your treatment team about how long you should have testing.

Your health care provider may also order imaging when treatment ends. Imaging of the chest and of any areas where cancer has spread is recommended. These scans will serve as a baseline to compare against future imaging results. You may continue to get scans of the site where the primary tumor was. How often depends on how likely the cancer is to return.

Widespread cancer

If the metastases are in many organs, the goal of care is palliative. Palliative care, also called supportive care, does not try to cure the cancer. It's used to relieve pain and discomfort, to reduce symptoms caused by the cancer, and to extend life. Palliative treatment options include:

- Systemic drug therapy (see **Guides 1** and **2**)
- Radiation
- Surgery
- Observation (if you have no symptoms)
- Supportive care
- Ablation procedures
- Embolization (for tumors not in the lungs)

Systemic drug therapy, radiation therapy, and surgery may reduce cancer symptoms by stopping or slowing tumor growth. Other options include ablation and embolization.

Follow-up care, including imaging, for widespread metastatic disease is individualized. Talk with your health care provider about how often you may need imaging and what other care to expect.

Supportive care

Supportive care helps improve your quality of life during and after cancer treatment. The goal is to prevent or manage side effects and symptoms, like pain and cancer-related fatigue. It also addresses the mental, social, and spiritual concerns faced by those with cancer.

Supportive care is available to everyone with cancer and their families, not just those at the end of life. Palliative care is another name for supportive care.

Supportive care can also help with:

- Making treatment decisions
- Coordinating your care
- Paying for care
- Planning for advanced care and end of life

If cancer returns

A recurrence is the return of cancer after a cancer-free period. Treatment options depend on the location of the new growth. If sarcoma returns to the area where it started, it's called local recurrence. Local recurrence is often treated as if it were newly diagnosed.

If the cancer returns and spreads to areas far from where it started, it's called distant recurrence. The cancer is metastatic. Treatment for metastatic disease is based on whether the new cancer growth is:

- Only in one organ
- In the same specific region or found in lymph nodes
- Widespread

If the cancer has **returned to only one organ** and the tumor is small, surgery to remove the metastatic tumor (metastasectomy) is often recommended, especially for lung tumors. Systemic drug therapy and possibly radiation therapy may be given before or after surgery.

Other recommended options for recurrence in one organ include:

- Radiation with or without systemic drug therapy
- Ablation procedures
- Embolization procedures (for tumors not in the lungs)
- Observation

If cancer returns to the same specific region and is **found in lymph nodes**, a regional lymph node dissection is recommended. This is surgery to remove these lymph nodes from your body. Surgery might be followed by radiation therapy. If radiation therapy is planned, systemic drug therapy may also be given.

The cancer may return to areas far from where it started. If the cancer is **widespread**, the main goal of care isn't to cure the cancer but to control its growth, extend your life, and make you more comfortable. This care could include:

- Systemic drug therapy (see **Guides 1** and **2**)
- Destroying metastatic tumors with radiation therapy
- Surgery
- Observation (if you don't have symptoms)
- Supportive care
- Ablation procedures
- Embolization procedures (for tumors not in the lungs)

Key points

- Most stage 1 and 2 sarcomas in the limbs, outer torso, head, or neck can be treated with surgery.
- For stage 3 and non-metastatic stage 4 sarcomas, surgery may come first, followed by radiation therapy or chemoradiation. Or, radiation therapy and/or systemic drug therapy may be given first to shrink the tumor.
- If surgery isn't possible, other treatment is given. This could include radiation therapy, chemoradiation, systemic drug therapy, or isolated limb infusion.
- If the limb will not function after surgery, amputation is sometimes the only option. Your treatment team will consider advances in limb reconstruction.
- Local therapies and/or systemic drug therapy will be considered to treat metastatic tumors. Observation may also be an option.
- The goal of care for widespread metastatic cancer is to control its growth and improve comfort and quality of life.
- Treatment for recurrence is based on the extent and location of the cancer.

Questions to ask

- Does any option offer a cure or long-term cancer control?
- What are the side effects of the treatments?
- How do I get a second opinion?
- How long do I have to decide about treatment, and is there a social worker or someone who can help me decide?

5
Sarcomas inside the abdomen

Soft tissue sarcomas found in organs inside the chest, abdomen, or pelvis are usually treated with surgery. Together, these areas are called the inner trunk or abdomen.

Organs found in the inner abdomen include the adrenal glands, aorta, kidneys, pancreas, rectum, stomach, and colon.

Liposarcoma and leiomyosarcoma are the most common types of soft tissue sarcoma found in the inner abdomen.

Tumors in the inner abdomen tend to grow very large before causing symptoms. They tend to push against or invade nearby structures such as veins and arteries. The size of the tumor and how close it is to major blood vessels may make surgery difficult.

A biopsy is needed to confirm soft tissue sarcoma in the abdomen.

Removable with surgery

When possible, surgery is recommended for soft tissue sarcomas in the inner abdomen. For sarcomas thought likely to return and/or spread, treatment may be given before surgery. This could involve radiation therapy or systemic drug therapy (chemotherapy, immunotherapy, or targeted therapy).

Organs of the inner abdomen include the kidneys, stomach, intestines, and pancreas.

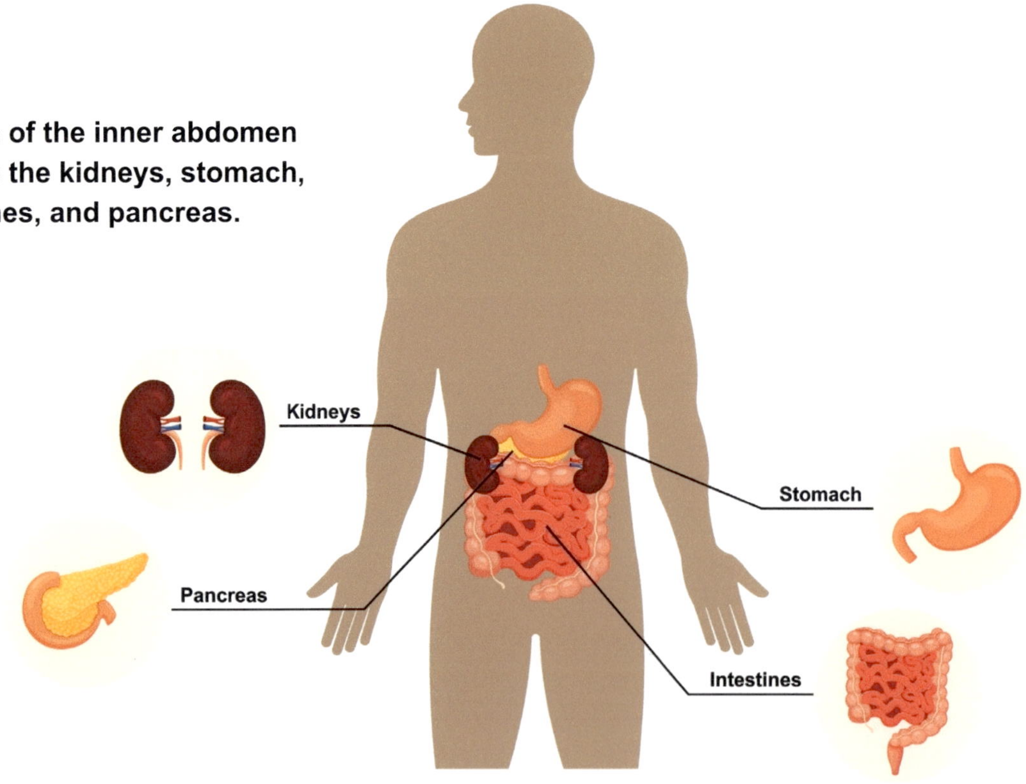

If treatment before surgery is being considered, an image-guided core needle biopsy is needed. An experienced sarcoma pathologist should review the biopsy samples.

If systemic drug therapy before surgery is planned, the drug(s) used will depend on the subtype of soft tissue sarcoma. Preferred systemic drug therapies for general soft tissue sarcoma are listed in **Guide 1** on page 29. Preferred systemic drug therapies for specific tumor types are listed in **Guide 2** on page 30.

After surgery, a pathologist examines the surgical margin for cancer cells. Depending on the results, more treatment may be needed. For any sarcoma thought to be at high risk of spreading, systemic drug therapy will be considered after surgery.

The best possible surgical outcome is called complete resection or negative margin. It means that no cancer cells were found in the surgical margin. If achieved, additional therapy may **not** be needed after surgery.

If the surgeon removes the tumor but cancer cells remain in the margin, it's a positive margin. This can happen when the tumor is close to important structures, like large blood vessels or nerves.

Some people with positive margins or a very narrow negative margin after surgery may benefit from radiation therapy.

If the tumor wasn't completely removed with surgery, a second surgery to remove the remaining cancer may be an option. This is generally only considered if complete removal is thought to be possible. You should also be healthy enough to have the surgery.

Follow-up care

When treatment is over, you'll have tests to look for signs of recurrence. Testing includes physical exams and imaging. For imaging, CT is generally preferred for sarcomas in these areas. MRI is also a recommended option. In some cases, PET may be combined with CT.

Imaging and a physical exam are recommended every 3 to 6 months for the first 3 years after treatment. For the following 2 years, testing is recommended every 6 months. After that, testing is recommended once per year.

If the cancer is likely to spread to the lungs, you may also get imaging tests of your chest.

Unremovable with surgery or stage 4

A tumor that can't be safely removed with surgery is called unremovable or unresectable. These include tumors that involve vital structures and tumors whose removal could cause complications or death.

Overall health also plays a role. You should be healthy enough to have major abdominal surgery.

Stage 4 tumors can be any size and any grade. Stage 4 cancer has spread to distant areas or, much less commonly, to nearby lymph nodes.

If the tumor is slow-growing and not causing symptoms, observation without treatment is one recommended option.

Sometimes an unremovable tumor can become removable. An attempt might be made to shrink the tumor using systemic drug therapy, radiation therapy, ablation, and/or embolization. Imaging tests will be used to see if the tumor has shrunk and if surgery is now possible.

If the tumor becomes removable, see *Removable with surgery* on page 36. If the tumor stays unresectable or gets worse, options include:

- Trying a different systemic drug therapy
- Trying radiation therapy to ease discomfort (palliative care)
- Getting supportive care

Supportive care doesn't try to cure cancer, but to relieve discomfort. Systemic drug therapy or radiation therapy may reduce cancer symptoms by stopping or slowing tumor growth.

If cancer returns

The return of cancer after a cancer-free period is called recurrence.

Surgery is recommended for any recurrent cancer growth that appears to be removable. After surgery, you may have radiation therapy or systemic drug therapy to reduce the risk of cancer growing back again.

In some cases, radiation therapy or systemic drug therapy is given before surgery. This helps shrink the tumor before surgery to make it more manageable. Systemic drug therapy before surgery is only considered if there's a high risk that the recurrence will spread. It's not recommended for low-grade tumors.

If the new cancer growth can't be removed with surgery, see *Unremovable with surgery or stage 4*.

Key points

- When possible, surgery is recommended for soft tissue sarcomas inside the abdomen. If surgery removes all of the tumor, it's called complete resection.
- For tumors expected to return and/or spread, radiation therapy or systemic drug therapy may be given first.
- Observation without treatment is a recommended option if the tumor is slow-growing and not causing symptoms.
- Systemic drug therapy and/or radiation therapy may be used before surgery to try to shrink the tumor.
- If the tumor is unremovable or it grows, options include a different systemic drug therapy, palliative radiation therapy, and supportive care.
- Radiation therapy or systemic drug therapy may be given after surgery to reduce the risk of cancer returning.

Questions to ask

- How will you know if treatment is working?
- What are the chances of the cancer returning?
- What follow-up care is needed after treatment?
- Will I be able to work while I'm undergoing treatment?

We want your feedback!

Our goal is to provide helpful and easy-to-understand information on cancer. Take our survey to let us know what we got right and what we could do better.
NCCN.org/patients/feedback

6
Desmoid tumors

Desmoid tumors are non-cancerous growths. They are treated like cancer, even though they do not spread through the body. These tumors are usually observed or treated with systemic drug therapy.

Not all tumors are cancerous. Desmoid tumors, also known as aggressive fibromatosis or desmoid-type fibromatosis, aren't considered cancerous because they do not spread in the body. But they can grow larger in the area where they start and cause symptoms.

If they return after treatment, they'll return to the same area as the first tumor.

Testing

Your health care provider will ask about your health history and perform a physical exam. A sample of the tumor will also be removed for testing.

Imaging of the tumor may also be needed. Either CT or MRI is recommended.

Hereditary syndromes

Desmoid tumors often occur for unknown reasons. However, some rare syndromes increase the risk of cancer and desmoid tumors. This includes familial adenomatous polyposis (FAP), described in *Chapter 1: About soft tissue sarcoma*.

Observation

Many newly diagnosed desmoid tumors should be observed without treatment, if the tumor is stable and not causing pain.

The tumor is monitored using CT or MRI scans every 3 months to start. Your imaging schedule will depend on the location of the tumor, the risk of progression to cancer, and any symptoms of progression. More frequent imaging may be needed if you have symptoms or if the tumor is near important body structures.

If the tumor is causing pain or other symptoms, systemic drug therapy may be an option. This depends on where the tumor is in the body and the safety of the drug.

If the desmoid tumor worsens somewhat but your symptoms aren't bad, your health care provider may recommend continuing observation. If growth continues and causes severe symptoms or problems, you'll need treatment. See *Treatment* on the next page.

Large tumors that are causing problems will be treated based on the location of the tumor, if it's causing pain, or if it interferes with movement.

Treatment

Treatment for desmoid tumors often includes systemic drug therapy and/or ablation. Surgery and radiation therapy are less commonly used. Each of these is discussed in more detail next. The best treatment(s) for you will depend on the location of the tumor.

Systemic drug therapy

Different types of systemic drug therapy are used to treat desmoid tumors. Options include chemotherapy and targeted therapies. Recommended systemic therapies for desmoid tumors are listed in **Guide 3**.

Treatment might also include nonsteroidal anti-inflammatory drugs (NSAIDs). NSAIDs help reduce fever, swelling, pain, and redness. A common over-the-counter NSAID is ibuprofen (Advil), for example.

Sulindac (Clinoril) and celecoxib (Celebrex) are NSAIDs that are commonly prescribed for people with symptoms. Celecoxib can cause heart issues or put those with heart issues at greater risk for side effects.

Guide 3
Systemic drug therapy for desmoid tumors

Drug name (in alphabetical order)	How it's given	Type of drug
Doxorubicin with or without dacarbazine	infusion	chemotherapy
Imatinib (Gleevec)	pill	targeted therapy
Liposomal doxorubicin (Doxil)	infusion	chemotherapy
Methotrexate and vinblastine	infusion	chemotherapy
Methotrexate and vinorelbine	infusion	targeted therapy
Nirogacestat (Ogsiveo)	pill	targeted therapy
Pazopanib (Votrient)	pill	targeted therapy
Sorafenib (Nexavar)	pill	targeted therapy

Thermal ablation

Thermal ablation uses extreme cold or extreme heat to destroy desmoid tumors. It can help control the size of the tumor. Types of ablation include radiofrequency ablation (RFA) and cryotherapy.

These procedures are typically done at specialty hospitals or health care centers that specialize in treating desmoid tumors.

Surgery

Desmoid tumors are hard to completely remove because they're hard to see. They also frequently grow back after surgery.

Surgery might not be considered if there is a risk of serious complications. It may be too dangerous based on the tumor location or your overall health. For these reasons, surgery is generally not the first treatment unless agreed upon by a team of experts.

If surgery is planned and the results are very good, it's called a complete resection. Observation is recommended next.

If microscopic desmoid tumor cells remain after surgery, options include another surgery or radiation therapy to kill leftover desmoid tumor cells, or observation.

If much of the desmoid tumor could not be removed, options include:

- Radiation therapy
- Systemic drug therapy
- Ablation procedures
- Observation

If these treatments don't remove all of the tumor, radical surgery may be considered. Radical surgery involves removing large areas of tissue and/or organs affected by the tumor.

The main goal of treatment is to maintain function. Amputation is rarely considered.

Radiation therapy

In general, radiation therapy is not a preferred treatment for desmoid tumors as it can increase risk for developing a cancer in the future. But when it is used, it is generally only recommended for desmoid tumors in the limbs (arms and legs), outer torso, head, neck, abdominal wall, pelvis, trunk, and chest cavity.

It's not recommended for desmoid tumors in the abdomen, except under special circumstances. Organs in the inner abdomen include the adrenal glands, aorta, kidneys, ureters, part of the pancreas, rectum, and parts of the stomach and colon.

Follow-up care

After treatment, you'll be monitored for symptoms. A change in symptoms may be a sign of tumor growth. Report any new or worsening symptoms to your health care provider.

Follow-up tests are used to see if the desmoid tumor is growing or has returned.

Imaging

Imaging with CT or MRI every 3 to 6 months for 3 years is recommended. After that, imaging is done every 6 months for 2 years. Depending on the location of the tumor, ultrasound may also be used for long-term follow-up.

Rehabilitation

You should receive rehabilitation services if needed. This may include occupational and/or physical therapy.

Key points

- Desmoid tumors (also called aggressive fibromatoses) are persistent, non-cancerous growths.
- Many newly diagnosed desmoid tumors can be observed without treatment. The tumor is monitored with imaging tests.
- If the tumor is causing pain or other symptoms, systemic drug therapy may be an option.
- If the cancer grows and causes severe symptoms or problems, treatment for progression is needed.
- Treatment for desmoid tumors could include systemic drug therapy, surgery, radiation therapy, and/or ablation.
- Surgery usually isn't the first treatment unless agreed upon by a team of experts.
- In general, radiation therapy is not recommended for desmoid tumors in the abdomen or torso.

Questions to ask

- Will I need any accommodation to continue to work during treatment?
- Does this hospital or cancer center offer the best treatment for me?
- Do I have a choice of when to begin treatment? How long will treatment last?
- Will my insurance cover the treatment you're recommending?

7 Rhabdomyosarcoma

Rhabdomyosarcoma (RMS) is more common in children than in adults. This type of soft tissue sarcoma usually starts in cells that develop into skeletal muscle.

Rhabdomyosarcoma (RMS) is a rare type of sarcoma of skeletal muscle. Skeletal muscles are those that you can control or move, such as your arms and legs.

RMS can also be found in parts of the body that don't normally have skeletal muscle, such as the reproductive system or the base of the skull.

Before you are born, cells called rhabdomyoblasts form in your body. These cells eventually become skeletal muscle.

But in rare cases, rhabdomyoblasts develop into RMS instead.

RMS is more common in children because it starts in rhabdomyoblasts, which are more present in children.

Risk factors for RMS include Li-Fraumeni syndrome and neurofibromatosis type 1 (NF1).

Skeletal muscles

Skeletal muscles are usually attached to bones of your skeleton. These are muscles you can control or move.

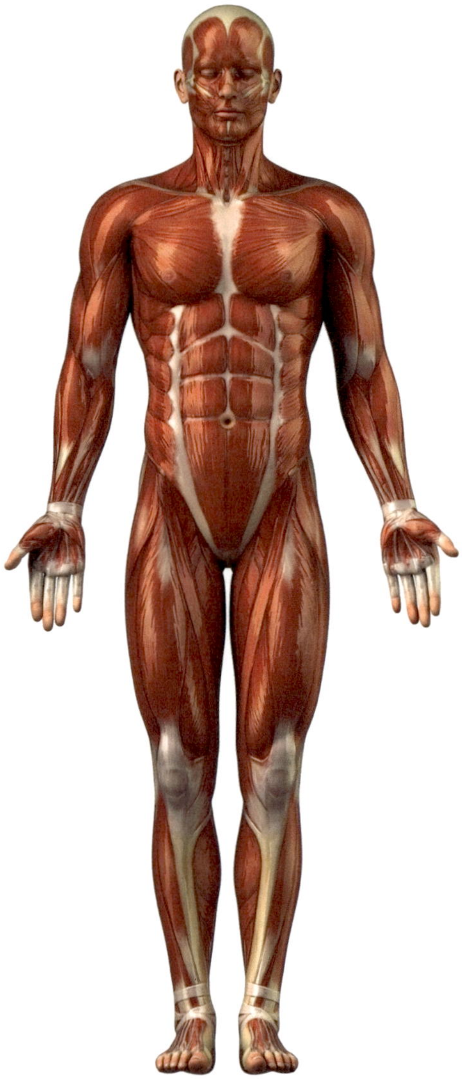

RMS in children

The type of RMS mostly seen in children is called non-pleomorphic RMS. It includes the following subtypes:

- Alveolar
- Embryonal
- Spindle cell/sclerosing

Alveolar RMS is often found in skeletal muscle of the legs and arms, but can be found in the torso, head, and neck. It's more aggressive than embryonal RMS.

Embryonal RMS tends to occur in the head, neck, bladder, vagina, and in or around the prostate and testicles.

Spindle cell/sclerosing RMS includes tumors with *VGLL2*-related genetic fusions, bone tumors, and tumors with *MYOD1* genetic mutations. The *MYOD1* mutated tumors are the most aggressive.

Spindle cell/sclerosing rhabdomyosarcomas that are present at birth or that occur shortly after birth are often less aggressive than other rhabdomyosarcomas.

Treatment

NCCN experts strongly recommend seeking treatment at a cancer center experienced in treating non-pleomorphic RMS. Treatment planning should involve a pediatric oncologist as well as medical, radiation, and surgical oncologists.

Treatment often involves a combination of surgery, systemic drug therapy, and radiation therapy.

The following chemotherapy combinations are preferred for non-pleomorphic RMS:

- Vincristine, dactinomycin, and cyclophosphamide
- Vincristine, dactinomycin, and ifosfamide

If treatment with these combinations is not possible, there are other recommended options for systemic drug therapy.

RMS in adults

In adults, pleomorphic RMS tends to grow quickly.

The most common areas in which pleomorphic RMS forms are the limbs, torso wall, reproductive system, or urinary system. The urinary system includes the kidneys, bladder, urethra, and ureters.

The outlook for pleomorphic RMS is not good. Not enough clinical research has been done on this type of RMS. This means there are little data on the best treatment for adults with RMS.

At this time, pleomorphic RMS is treated like high-grade undifferentiated pleomorphic sarcoma (UPS). Treatment may involve surgery, radiation therapy, and one of the systemic drug therapies seen in **Guides 1** and **2**.

Key points

- Rhabdomyosarcoma (RMS) is a rare type of sarcoma of skeletal muscle.
- RMS can also be found in parts of the body that don't normally have skeletal muscle.
- RMS is more common in children because it starts in premature cells called rhabdomyoblasts. RMS in children is called non-pleomorphic RMS. It includes embryonal, alveolar, and spindle cell/sclerosing subtypes.
- Risk factors for RMS include Li-Fraumeni syndrome and neurofibromatosis type 1 (NF1).
- Treatment should be planned by a team of specialists at a center experienced in treating non-pleomorphic RMS.
- Those with RMS often require more than one type of cancer treatment, including surgery, radiation therapy, and/or systemic drug therapy.
- Pleomorphic RMS is a rare, fast-growing sarcoma that occurs mostly in older adults.

Questions to ask

- What are the possible complications and side effects of treatment?
- Is a clinical trial an option for me?
- What will happen if I do nothing?
- Are you suggesting options other than what NCCN recommends? If yes, why?

8

Atypical lipomatous tumor/ Well-differentiated liposarcoma

Atypical lipomatous tumor (ALT)/ well-differentiated liposarcoma (WDLS) is one of five major types of liposarcoma. Liposarcoma is a rare soft tissue sarcoma that starts in fat cells.

This complex name reflects tumors that look the same through the microscope but act differently depending on how they form. As tumors evolve from normal tissue, they transform from normal cells into less organized and recognizable cells. This process is called "differentiation." Tumors that are less recognizable as their original selves are called "dedifferentiated."

Tumors that develop in the arms or legs may return to the same area after a very long time (years to decades), and are called atypical lipomatous tumors. Sometimes they become simpler in structure, but not often, and even less often, they cause death. Some sarcoma health care providers prefer the name "ALT" for these tumors when they occur in the arms or legs.

Tumors that develop in the torso often return to the same area, often become dedifferentiated, and sometimes (years to decades later) can cause death, and are called well-differentiated liposarcoma. Most sarcoma health care providers prefer the name "WDLS" for these tumors. They're generally more aggressive than ALT.

While rare, ALT/WDLS can transform over time into a related type of liposarcoma called dedifferentiated liposarcoma. Lab tests or imaging scans can diagnose the features signaling this change.

Dedifferentiated liposarcoma usually grows faster than ALT/WDLS. It's also more likely to return after treatment and/or spread to distant areas of the body (metastasize).

Treatment

Limbs, abdominal wall, or torso

Treatment for ALT/WDLS that forms in these areas depends on whether there is evidence of dedifferentiation. If there isn't evidence of dedifferentiation or higher-grade sarcoma, surgery alone to remove the tumor is recommended.

After surgery, some tumor cells may be found in the normal tissue surrounding the tumor. But more treatment is not typically needed because these tumors don't usually spread to other areas of the body. If the tumor returns, either observation or another surgery is recommended.

Radiation therapy is not always recommended for atypical lipomatous tumors because they are considered "indolent" tumors, which means that they grow slowly and are generally not aggressive. See *Follow-up* on the next page for information on surveillance after surgery.

If there are signs of dedifferentiation, the same treatment used for other soft tissue sarcomas that form in these areas is recommended. For more information, see *Chapter 4: Sarcomas in the limbs, outer torso, head, or neck*.

Inner abdomen or scrotum

For ALT/WDLS that forms in the inner abdomen or scrotum, treatment is not guided by whether there is dedifferentiation. In that case, the same treatment used for other soft tissue sarcomas that form in these areas is recommended. See Chapter 5 of this guide, *Sarcomas inside the abdomen*.

Follow-up

Surveillance after treatment includes physical exams and imaging of the area where the tumor formed.

A physical exam is recommended every 6 to 12 months for the first 2 years after treatment. After that, 1 exam per year is recommended. But you may need them more or less often, depending on the risk of the cancer returning.

How often imaging is needed will be based on where the tumor started. Your health care provider will consider the location (how easily it can be examined without imaging) and how likely the cancer is to return.

Imaging of the chest to check if the cancer has spread isn't recommended, unless dedifferentiation occurred.

Key points

- Atypical lipomatous tumor (ALT) is a sarcoma that develops in the arms or legs, and takes a very long time to return.
- Well-differentiated liposarcoma (WDLS) is a more aggressive sarcoma compared to ALT that develops in the torso and can cause death.
- Treatment of ALT/WDLS depends on whether there is evidence of dedifferentiation. If there is, then the cancer will be treated more aggressively.
- If the cells are well-differentiated, then surgery alone is recommended for treating ALT/WDLS.
- You may get imaging of your chest to monitor for cancer spreading to the lungs.

Questions to ask

- Does any option offer a cure or long-term cancer control?
- What are the side effects of the treatments?
- How do I get a second opinion?

9

Other resources

Want to learn more? Here's how you can get additional help.

What else to know

This book can help you improve your cancer care. It plainly explains expert recommendations and suggests questions to ask your care team. But it's not the only resource that you have.

You're welcome to receive as much information and help as you need. Many people are interested in learning more about:

- The details of their health and treatment
- Being a part of a care team
- Getting financial help
- Finding a sarcoma expert
- Coping with health problems

What else to do

Your health care center can help you with the next steps. They often have on-site resources to help meet your needs and find answers to your questions. Health care centers can also inform you of resources in your community.

In addition to help from your providers, the resources listed in the next section provide support for many people like yourself. Look through the list and visit the provided websites to learn more about these organizations.

Where to get help

Cancer*Care*
cancercare.org

Clear Cell Sarcoma Foundation
Clearcellsarcoma.org

Desmoid Tumors Research Foundation
DTRF.org

GRACE
cancergrace.org

Imerman Angels
imermanangels.org

Leiomyosarcoma Support & Direct Research Foundation
lmsdr.org

National Coalition for Cancer Survivorship
canceradvocacy.org

National LeioMyoSarcoma Foundation
nlmsf.org

Northwest Sarcoma Foundation
nwsarcoma.org

Sarcoma Foundation of America
curesarcoma.org

Stupid Cancer
Stupidcancer.org

TargetCancer Foundation
Targetcancer.org

The Alan B. Slifka Foundation
Slifkafoundation.org

The Life Raft Group
liferaftgroup.org

The Paula Takacs Foundation
paulatakacsfoundation.org

Triage Cancer
Triagecancer.org

Questions to ask

- Are you board-certified? If yes, in what area?
- Is treatment of soft tissue sarcoma a major part of your practice?
- How many people with my type of soft tissue sarcoma have you treated?
- Will you be consulting with other experts to discuss my care? Whom will you consult?
- How many of your patients have had complications? What were the complications?

Let us know what you think!

Please take a moment to complete an online survey about the NCCN Guidelines for Patients.
NCCN.org/patients/response

Words to know

ablation
A treatment that destroys very small tumors with heat, cold, lasers, or chemicals. Also called ablative therapy.

biopsy
A procedure that removes fluid or tissue samples to be tested for disease.

brachytherapy
A treatment with radiation from an object placed near or in the tumor. Also called internal radiation.

chemoembolization
A cancer treatment with chemotherapy-coated beads that block blood supply to tumors.

chemoradiation
Treatment with a combination of chemotherapy and radiation therapy.

chemotherapy
Drugs that kill cancer cells by damaging or disrupting the making of the genetic code.

computed tomography (CT)
A test that uses x-rays from many angles to make a picture of the insides of the body.

contrast
A substance put into your body to make clearer pictures during imaging tests.

core needle biopsy
A procedure that removes tissue samples with a hollow needle. Also called core biopsy.

cryotherapy
A type of ablation therapy that kills cancer cells by freezing them.

desmoid tumor
A non-cancerous mass of fibrous cells that grows into nearby tissue and rarely spreads to distant sites. Also known as aggressive fibromatosis.

distant recurrence
Cancer that has come back after treatment and is found in a part of the body far from the first (primary) tumor.

embolization
A treatment that cuts off blood supply to tumors with beads inserted into an artery.

external beam radiation therapy (EBRT)
A cancer treatment with radiation delivered from a machine outside the body.

familial adenomatous polyposis (FAP)
A hereditary condition that causes many abnormal growths (polyps) to form in the bowel. Increases the risk of sarcoma.

Gardner syndrome
A hereditary syndrome that causes bowel polyps, abnormal bony growths, and skin and soft tissue tumors. A type of familial adenomatous polyposis (FAP).

grade
A rating of how quickly a cancer is expected to grow, based on how abnormal the cancer cells look under a microscope.

histology
The structure of cells, tissue, and organs as viewed under a microscope.

immunotherapy
A treatment with drugs that help the body find and destroy cancer cells.

intensity-modulated radiation therapy
Treatment with radiation that uses small beams of different strengths based on the thickness of the tissue. A type of EBRT.

intraoperative radiation therapy
Radiation therapy given during surgery.

isolated limb infusion/perfusion
A method of giving cancer drugs directly into the bloodstream of a limb (arm or leg).

Li-Fraumeni syndrome
A health condition passed down in a family that increases the chance of getting sarcoma and other cancers.

local recurrence
Cancer that returns to the same general area after treatment.

lymph node
A small, bean-shaped, disease-fighting structure.

lymph node dissection
Surgery to remove one or more lymph nodes.

magnetic resonance imaging (MRI)
A test that uses radio waves and powerful magnets to make pictures of the insides of the body.

medical oncologist
A doctor who's an expert in cancer drugs.

metastasectomy
Surgery to remove tumors that formed far from the first site of cancer. Used to reduce cancer burden and to ease symptoms.

metastasis
The spread of cancer cells from the first (primary) tumor to a new site.

neurofibromatosis
A rare genetic condition that causes tumors to grow on nerves. Increases the risk of soft tissue sarcoma.

observation
A period of testing for changes in cancer status while not receiving treatment.

occupational therapist
An expert in helping people live life unaided.

oncology surgeon
A doctor who's an expert in operations that remove cancer.

palliative care
Health care that includes symptom relief but not cancer treatment. Also sometimes called supportive care.

pathologist
A doctor who's an expert in testing cells and tissue to find disease.

physical therapist
An expert in helping people move better.

positron emission tomography (PET)
A test that uses radioactive material to see the shape and function of body parts.

primary tumor
The first and main tumor.

progression
The growth or spread of cancer after being tested or treated.

radiation oncologist
A doctor who's an expert in treating cancer with radiation.

radiation therapy
A local treatment that uses high-energy rays or related approaches to kill cancer cells.

radiofrequency ablation
A treatment that destroys cancer cells by heating them with high-energy radio waves.

radiologist
A doctor who's an expert in interpreting imaging tests.

recurrence
The return or worsening of cancer after a period of improvement.

resectable
Cancer that can be completely removed with surgery.

torso
The body space in front of the spine in the lower trunk.

rhabdomyosarcoma (RMS)
A type of soft tissue sarcoma that starts in the cells that normally develop into skeletal muscle.

sarcoma
A cancer of bone or soft tissue cells.

stereotactic body radiation therapy
Radiation therapy given in higher doses to smaller areas over 1 to 5 sessions of treatment.

supportive care
Health care that includes symptom relief but not cancer treatment. Also called palliative care.

surgical margin
The normal-looking tissue around the edge of a tumor removed during surgery.

targeted therapy
A drug treatment that impedes the growth process specific to cancer cells.

thoracic surgeon
A doctor who's an expert in operating on organs inside the chest.

ultrasound
A test that uses sound waves to take pictures of the insides of the body.

unresectable
Cancer that can't be removed with surgery.

x-ray
A noninvasive imaging test that uses a small amount of radiation. Also called a plain radiograph.

NCCN Contributors

This patient guide is based on the NCCN Clinical Practice Guidelines in Oncology (NCCN Guidelines®) for Soft Tissue Sarcoma, Version 1.2025. It was adapted, reviewed, and published with help from the following people:

Dorothy A. Shead, MS
Senior Director
Patient Information Operations

Tim Rinehart, MS
Medical Writer, Patient Information

Lisa Diehl
Production Layout Artist

The NCCN Clinical Practice Guidelines in Oncology (NCCN Guidelines®) for Soft Tissue Sarcoma, Version 1.2025 were developed by the following NCCN Panel Members:

Margaret von Mehren, MD/Chair
Fox Chase Cancer Center

John M. Kane, III, MD/Vice-Chair
Roswell Park Comprehensive Cancer Center

Samantha A. Armstrong, MD
Indiana University Melvin and Bren Simon Comprehensive Cancer Center

Tessa Balach, MD
The UChicago Medicine Comprehensive Cancer Center

Andrew J. Bishop, MD
The University of Texas MD Anderson Cancer Center

Darya Buehler, MD
Moffitt Cancer Center

Janai Carr-Ascher, MD, PhD
UC Davis Comprehensive Cancer Center

*Edwin Choy, MD, PhD
Mass General Cancer Center

Cara Cipriano, MD, MSc
Abramson Cancer Center at the University of Pennsylvania

*Mary Connolly, MSW
The Ohio State University Comprehensive Cancer Center - James Cancer Hospital and Solove Research Institute

Amanda Dann, MD
UT Southwestern Simmons Comprehensive Cancer Center

Elizabeth J. Davis, MD
Vanderbilt-Ingram Cancer Center

Sarah Dry, MD
UCLA Jonsson Comprehensive Cancer Center

Vanessa Eulo, MD
O'Neal Comprehensive Cancer Center at UAB

Kristen N. Ganjoo, MD
Stanford Cancer Institute

Ricardo J. Gonzalez, MD
Moffitt Cancer Center

Pedro A. Hermida De Viveiros, MD
Robert H. Lurie Comprehensive Cancer Center of Northwestern University

*Ying J. Hitchcock, MD
Huntsman Cancer Institute at the University of Utah

Edward Kim, MD
Fred Hutchinson Cancer Center

Daniel Lefler, MD
Abramson Cancer Center at the University of Pennsylvania

David Liebner, MD
The Ohio State University Comprehensive Cancer Center - James Cancer Hospital and Solove Research Institute

*Martin McCarter, MD
University of Colorado Cancer Center

Sean V. McGarry, MD
Fred & Pamela Buffett Cancer Center

Nathan W. Mesko, MD
Case Comprehensive Cancer Center/ University Hospitals Seidman Cancer Center and Cleveland Clinic Taussig Cancer Institute

Christian Meyer, MD, PhD
Johns Hopkins Kimmel Cancer Center

Kambiz Motamedi, MD
UCLA Jonsson Comprehensive Cancer Center

Sujana Movva, MD
Memorial Sloan Kettering Cancer Center

Alberto S. Pappo, MD
St. Jude Children's Research Hospital/ The University of Tennessee Health Science Center

Seth M. Pollack, MD
Robert H. Lurie Comprehensive Cancer Center of Northwestern University

Matthew Poppe, MD
Huntsman Cancer Institute at the University of Utah

Richard F. Riedel, MD
Duke Cancer Institute

Steven Robinson, MBBS
Mayo Clinic Comprehensive Cancer Center

Scott Schuetze, MD, PhD
University of Michigan Rogel Cancer Center

Jason K. Sicklick, MD
UC San Diego Moores Cancer Center

*William Tseng, MD
City of Hope National Medical Center

Mia C. Weiss, MD
Siteman Cancer Center at Barnes-Jewish Hospital and Washington University School of Medicine

Melissa Zimel, MD
UCSF Helen Diller Family Comprehensive Cancer Center

NCCN

Mary Anne Bergman
Guidelines Coordinator

Zeenat Diwan, MS, PhD
Associate Scientist/Medical Writer

Lisa Hang, PhD
Manager, Clinical Content Processes

* Reviewed this patient guide. For disclosures, visit NCCN.org/disclosures.

NCCN Cancer Centers

Abramson Cancer Center
at the University of Pennsylvania
Philadelphia, Pennsylvania
800.789.7366 • pennmedicine.org/cancer

Case Comprehensive Cancer Center/
University Hospitals Seidman Cancer Center and
Cleveland Clinic Taussig Cancer Institute
Cleveland, Ohio
UH Seidman Cancer Center
800.641.2422 • uhhospitals.org/services/cancer-services
CC Taussig Cancer Institute
866.223.8100 • my.clevelandclinic.org/departments/cancer
Case CCC
216.844.8797 • case.edu/cancer

City of Hope National Medical Center
Duarte, California
800.826.4673 • cityofhope.org

Dana-Farber/Brigham and Women's Cancer Center |
Mass General Cancer Center
Boston, Massachusetts
877.442.3324 • youhaveus.org
617.726.5130 • massgeneral.org/cancer-center

Duke Cancer Institute
Durham, North Carolina
888.275.3853 • dukecancerinstitute.org

Fox Chase Cancer Center
Philadelphia, Pennsylvania
888.369.2427 • foxchase.org

Fred & Pamela Buffett Cancer Center
Omaha, Nebraska
402.559.5600 • unmc.edu/cancercenter

Fred Hutchinson Cancer Center
Seattle, Washington
206.667.5000 • fredhutch.org

Huntsman Cancer Institute at the University of Utah
Salt Lake City, Utah
800.824.2073 • healthcare.utah.edu/huntsmancancerinstitute

Indiana University Melvin and Bren Simon
Comprehensive Cancer Center
Indianapolis, Indiana
888.600.4822 • www.cancer.iu.edu

Johns Hopkins Kimmel Cancer Center
Baltimore, Maryland
410.955.8964
www.hopkinskimmelcancercenter.org

Mayo Clinic Comprehensive Cancer Center
Phoenix/Scottsdale, Arizona
Jacksonville, Florida
Rochester, Minnesota
480.301.8000 • Arizona
904.953.0853 • Florida
507.538.3270 • Minnesota
mayoclinic.org/cancercenter

Memorial Sloan Kettering Cancer Center
New York, New York
800.525.2225 • mskcc.org

Moffitt Cancer Center
Tampa, Florida
888.663.3488 • moffitt.org

O'Neal Comprehensive Cancer Center at UAB
Birmingham, Alabama
800.822.0933 • uab.edu/onealcancercenter

Robert H. Lurie Comprehensive Cancer Center
of Northwestern University
Chicago, Illinois
866.587.4322 • cancer.northwestern.edu

Roswell Park Comprehensive Cancer Center
Buffalo, New York
877.275.7724 • roswellpark.org

Siteman Cancer Center at Barnes-Jewish Hospital
and Washington University School of Medicine
St. Louis, Missouri
800.600.3606 • siteman.wustl.edu

St. Jude Children's Research Hospital/
The University of Tennessee Health Science Center
Memphis, Tennessee
866.278.5833 • stjude.org
901.448.5500 • uthsc.edu

Stanford Cancer Institute
Stanford, California
877.668.7535 • cancer.stanford.edu

The Ohio State University Comprehensive Cancer Center -
James Cancer Hospital and Solove Research Institute
Columbus, Ohio
800.293.5066 • cancer.osu.edu

The UChicago Medicine Comprehensive Cancer Center
Chicago, Illinois
773.702.1000 • uchicagomedicine.org/cancer

The University of Texas MD Anderson Cancer Center
Houston, Texas
844.269.5922 • mdanderson.org

UC Davis Comprehensive Cancer Center
Sacramento, California
916.734.5959 • 800.770.9261
health.ucdavis.edu/cancer

UC San Diego Moores Cancer Center
La Jolla, California
858.822.6100 • cancer.ucsd.edu

UCLA Jonsson Comprehensive Cancer Center
Los Angeles, California
310.825.5268 • uclahealth.org/cancer

UCSF Helen Diller Family
Comprehensive Cancer Center
San Francisco, California
800.689.8273 • cancer.ucsf.edu

University of Colorado Cancer Center
Aurora, Colorado
720.848.0300 • coloradocancercenter.org

University of Michigan Rogel Cancer Center
Ann Arbor, Michigan
800.865.1125 • rogelcancercenter.org

University of Wisconsin Carbone Cancer Center
Madison, Wisconsin
608.265.1700 • uwhealth.org/cancer

UT Southwestern Simmons
Comprehensive Cancer Center
Dallas, Texas
214.648.3111 • utsouthwestern.edu/simmons

Vanderbilt-Ingram Cancer Center
Nashville, Tennessee
877.936.8422 • vicc.org

Yale Cancer Center/Smilow Cancer Hospital
New Haven, Connecticut
855.4.SMILOW • yalecancercenter.org

share with us.

Take our survey and help make the NCCN Guidelines for Patients better for everyone!

NCCN.org/patients/comments

Index

Made in the USA
Monee, IL
12 September 2026

62980070R00038